HANDBOOK TO RECOGNIZE ADHESIVE ARACHNOIDITIS BY MAGNETIC RESONANCE IMAGING (MRI)

By

Forest Tennant, MPH, DrPH, MD

Published by the
Tennant Foundation
West Covina, California

Copyright© 2021 Tennant Foundation

All rights reserved. This book or any portion thereof may not be reproduced or used in any manner whatsoever without the express written permission of the publisher except for the use of brief quotations in a book review or scholarly journal.

ISBN: 9781955934152
Library of Congress Control Number: 2021925161

Ordering Information:

Special discounts are available on quantity purchases by corporations, associations, educators, and others. For details, contact one of the parties listed below.

U.S. trade bookstores and wholesalers: Please contact
Nancy Kriskovich Tel: (406)249-2002;
or email snkriskovich@gmail.com
Medical Research and Education Project
c/o Nancy Kriskovich
14 Hidden River Lane
Bigfork, MT 59911

All proceeds from the sale of this book will go to the Medical Research and Education Projects sponsored by the
TENNANT FOUNDATION.
336 ½ S. GLENDORA AVENUE
WEST COVINA, CA 91790-3060
A 501(c)(3) Non-profit Organization

ACKNOWLEDGEMENTS

TENNANT FOUNDATION BOARD OF DIRECTORS

Chairperson: Jerry Muszynski
President: Forest Tennant
Vice President: Miriam Tennant
Secretary: Kathy Clark Treasurer:
James Hetzel

BOARD MEMBERS

Doran Barnes
Steve Castillo
Sander De Wildt
Don Scheliga
Vicki Scheliga
Tony Song
Ken Yoho

MEDICAL RESEARCH AND EDUCATION COMMITTEE

Chairperson: Ingrid Hollis
Lynn Ashcraft
Donna Corley
K. Scott Guess, Pharm D
Ryle Holder, Pharm D
Denise Molohon
Rhonda Posey
Gary Snook

ACKNOWLEDGMENTS

This book could not have been researched and written without the technical assistance of Becky and Tom Marino and Nancy Kriskovich.

DEDICATION

This Handbook is dedicated to Antonio Aldrete MD and Sarah Fox MD who pioneered the association of clinical symptoms and history with the findings on myelograms and magnetic resonance imaging.

Disclaimer: The information in this handbook including the MRI images displayed are from participants in a "Research and Education Project" sponsored and financed by the Tennant Foundation, a non-profit 501C-3 organization. All participants had personal physicians. Participants and physicians voluntarily submitted MRIs for review as no participant was examined, charged a fee, prescribed any medication, and no medical records were developed on participants.

Table of Contents

AUTHOR'S NOTES 1
1. INTRODUCTION 3
2. WHO SHOULD HAVE A LUMBAR-SACRAL CONTRAST MRI? 5
3. TERMS AND DEFINITIONS 6
4. HOW LUMBAR SACRAL ADHESIVE ARACHNOIDITIS DEVELOPS ... 9
5. FRONTAL ILLUSTRATION OF THE CAUDA EQUINA NERVE ROOTS 10
6. FRONTAL PHOTOGRAPH OF NORMAL CAUDA EQUINA NERVE ROOTS. 11
7. LATERAL VIEW OF THE CAUDA EQUINA 12
8. ANATOMICAL AXIAL APPEARANCE OF THE SPINAL CANAL 13
9. NORMAL POSITIONS OF THE CAUDA EQUINA NERVE ROOTS: AXIAL VIEWS. 14
10. PHOTOGRAPHS OF NORMAL CAUDA EQUINA NERVE ROOTS: AXIAL VIEWS 16
11. NORMAL CONTRAST MRI IMAGE OF CAUDA EQUINA NERVE ROOTS: AXIAL VIEW 18
12. ABNORMALITIES FOUND ON AXIAL CONTRAST MRIs 19
13. ABNORMALITIES FOUND ON LATERAL CONTRAST MRIs 20
14. BASIC APPEARANCE OF ADHESIVE ARACHNOIDITIS: SINGLE CLUMP 22
15. BASIC APPEARANCE OF ADHESIVE ARACHNOIDITIS: MULTIPLE CLUMPS 23
16. PROCESS AND TIME FRAME FOR DEVELOPMENT OF AA 24
17. CLINICAL PROFILE OF ABNORMAL EXAMPLES 26
18. EXAMPLES OF NORMAL MRI AXIAL VIEWS 27
19. EXAMPLES OF ABNORMAL AXIAL VIEW MRIs 29
20. NORMAL LATERAL VIEW MRI 43
21. EXAMPLES OF ABNORMAL LATERAL VIEW MRIs 44
22. SUMMARY 59

AUTHOR'S NOTES

Adhesive arachnoiditis (AA) is an intraspinal, canal inflammatory disorder. It occurs when some cauda equina nerve roots become glued to the inside of the spinal canal covering due to inflammation and adhesions. The term arachnoid is applied because it is the layer of the spinal canal covering inside the outer dural layer.

Approximately, five years ago the Tennant Foundation launched a Research and Education Project on Adhesive Arachnoiditis (hereafter AA), because it had become clear that this disorder was fast emerging as a major cause of severe intractable pain and significant disability. This emergence has occurred rather suddenly and unexpected. It can arguably be called a new public health issue. The mission of the Project is to bring diagnosis and treatment of this horrible condition to every community. A major part of this Project has been to develop a clinical profile of AA and interpret magnetic resonance imaging (MRI) from cases with typical symptoms of AA. To this end we have reviewed over 600 MRIs from 48 different countries.

The major goal of this handbook is to help medical practitioners recognize and initiate treatment of AA as early as possible. Like all chronic medical conditions, the earlier the diagnosis and treatment, the better the outcome.

Although there is no specific treatment for AA, it is a painful inflammatory disorder of the spinal canal. Like rheumatoid arthritis in the days before modern biologics, it responds to some anti-inflammatory, nutritional, physical, and pain control measures.

I wish to note that our findings support and are in consonance with the few, but excellent clinical publications and books that have been written about AA. This includes the pioneering, first efforts of the famed British neurosurgeon, Sir Victor Horsley. In 1909, he identified inflammation in the arachnoid-dural covering of the spinal canal and called the condition "chronic spinal meningitis."[12] To be saluted also is the seminal work of Samuel Harvey MD, who first found, in 1926, that adhesions between the spinal canal covering (meninges) and nerve roots, spinal cord, or brain were the real culprits that caused pain, disability, and interruption of spinal fluid flow.[9]

In summary, about a century ago, it was known that inflammation and adhesions inside the spinal canal are the two pathologic causes of AA. The great advances of contrast MRIs differentiates spinal fluid from solid tissue allowing us to visualize the inflammatory-adhesive changes first identified by Horsley and Harvey.[17]

I wish to thank my radiologist friends who encouraged me to embark on the MRI project and to develop this handbook. Five years ago, no one including me knew a lot about AA much less what it looked like on MRI. Naturally as a non-radiologist, I had some trepidation about researching a radiology topic; however, one good radiology friend said to me, five years ago, "We radiologists know almost nothing about AA. To develop good radiologic knowledge, someone must first know the disease. You know the disease. You can identify the pictures." In my investigative journey I have discovered that some excellent articles on MRI images of AA have been published and have been extremely helpful.[2,4,5,11,13,14,17] I also wish to credit Dr. Antonio Aldrete who was a master at interpreting AA findings on MRI.[1] He was also the physician who initiated and mentored my involvement with AA, and whose enthusiasm, dedication, and care for these patients has compelled me to carry on his pioneering work.

1. INTRODUCTION

Adhesive arachnoiditis (AA) is an intraspinal canal inflammatory disorder that occurs when adhesions cause cauda equina nerve roots to become glued to the inside of the spinal canal covering (meninges).[1,3] Although the incidence and prevalence of AA is not precisely known, it has paralleled the rise of herniated or protruding intervertebral discs in the population.[11,13,15] Factors that have given rise to lower back pain and disc issues include sedentary lifestyle, lack of exercise, obesity, diabetes, contact sports, and workplace injuries. Most patients with AA have pre-existing disc issues prior to developing the disorder.[11,13,15] Attempts to treat protruding discs with invasive procedures including surgery and epidural corticosteroid injections have unfortunately helped accelerate the rise of AA.[5,8]

It is now known that degenerating discs are inflamed and the inflammation may spread to the arachnoid layer of the spinal canal covering (meninges) and cauda equina nerve roots.[13] Other causes of AA that have helped give rise to the increasing incidence and prevalence of AA include genetic connective tissue/collagen disorders of the Ehlers-Danlos Syndrome class, autoimmune disorders, trauma including punctures of the spinal canal covering, and infections by some viruses and bacteria including Lyme Disease.[10] Regardless of the precise cause of an individual case, AA of the lumbar-sacral spine is now common enough that all medical practitioners must be aware of it.

Contrast MRI technology, allows spinal fluid to be visually distinguished from solid tissues, making interpretation possible for the medical practitioner. Given the high prevalence of back pain in society, it is the author's opinion that every medical practitioner can and should be able to do basic interpretation of lumbar-sacral contrast MRIs. They don't need to be a radiologist to diagnose tumors in a chest xray or a fracture of a leg. The interpretation for diagnosis of AA on MRI is analogous to these obvious problems in that most cases are quite obvious.

This handbook does not cover cervical, thoracic, or brain AA since these cases are extremely rare and require separate diagnostic guidelines from the more common AA of the lumbar-sacral spine. This handbook does not portend to provide information on any other spinal column or canal disorder but focuses entirely on the intraspinal canal inflammatory disorder known as AA.

2. WHO SHOULD HAVE A LUMBAR-SACRAL CONTRAST MRI?

AA is a secondary disorder in that some disease process has to initiate inflammation in either the cauda equina nerve roots or the arachnoid-dura covering of the spinal canal. [1,3,4,5,8]

Persons with AA have a rather standard symptom profile which is reflected in the six symptoms/manifestations shown below. Symptoms result, from cauda equina nerve roots being trapped in a mass (or clump) that is inflamed and glued by adhesions to the inside of the arachnoid-dural covering of the spinal canal. The location of the nerve root entrapment is typically between lumbar four (L-4), and sacral two (S-2), as this is the area of the spinal column that typically has the most protruding, intervertebral discs. Nerve roots in this area connect to the intestine, bladder, sex organs, rectum, legs, and feet, and are, therefore, responsible for most of the symptoms of AA.

Symptoms that justify a contrast MRI should include a majority of these clinical manifestations:

>1. Constant back pain with stabbing or shooting pains into the buttocks, legs, or feet.
>
>2. Pain is lessened by standing or reclining.
>
>3. Difficulty starting, stopping, or holding urination and/or defecation.
>
>4. Burning or electrical shock sensations in the feet.
>
>5. Sensation of insects crawling or water dripping on the legs.
>
>6. Pain is increased by walking upstairs or lying flat on the back.

3. TERMS AND DEFINITIONS

Adhesive arachnoiditis: An intraspinal canal inflammatory disorder in which there is a clump or mass of cauda equina nerve roots that are glued by adhesions to the arachnoid-dural covering of the spinal canal.[3]

Adhesive arachnoiditis ossification: This term has been applied to cases that show calcification in the clump or mass of AA.[18]

Arachnoiditis-non-adhesive: Inflammation of the arachnoid layer of the spinal canal covering (meninges) without any nerve roots adhered to it. This condition cannot specifically be identified by MRI. It is a clinical diagnosis based on signs, symptoms, and laboratory tests.

Axial view: "Toe-to-Head" view or images of the cauda equina and spinal canal. It is a cross section or pictorial "slice" of the spinal canal.

Canal Dilation/Distortion: The normal circular contour of the spinal canal has lost its normal shape due to some pathologic process such as fibrosis, scarring, or loss of tensile strength.

Cauda equina: About two dozen nerve roots that emanate from the spinal cord at about the level of thoracic 12 (T-12) or lumbar 1 (L-1) and are suspended in spinal fluid.

Circular contour: Cauda equina nerve roots appear circular on the axial view of an MRI. Loss of circular contour represents edema, inflammation, or degeneration.

Clumping or coalescence: Multiple nerve roots have joined together due to inflammation and adhesion formation.

Contrast: The ability to distinguish spinal fluid by white

coloring from solid tissue which shows as varying shades of gray. This may be accomplished with intravenous dye or with high resolution imaging.

Disorganization: Displacement of nerve roots with distortion of their normal nerve root pattern.

Displacement: Some nerve roots are moved or located to an abnormal position on axial (toe-to-head) MRI images.

Empty sac: The lower lumbar and/or sacral spinal canal is dilated with no sign of nerve roots passing through the interior of the canal. The cause is nerve roots attached to the inside of the spinal canal covering rather than be free floating in the spinal fluid.

Lumbar levels: There are five lumbar vertebrae levels being designated L1 through L5, with L1 being the topmost vertebrae.

Meninges: This is the spinal canal covering in the lumbar-sacral region that primarily consists of an inside layer called arachnoid and an outer layer called the dura. The word "covering" is preferentially used in this handbook rather than meninges or theca to simplify understanding.

Peripheralization: Cauda equina nerve roots are glued by adhesions to the inside of the spinal canal cover. This finding is often called "empty sac" as the canal may look empty and be dilated on both axial and lateral views.

Sacral levels: Two sacral levels will be noted in this handbook. These vertebrae will be designated S1 and S2.

Sagittal View: This is the side or lateral MRI view of the spine.

Seepage: Spinal fluid that has leaked or seeped into tissues outside the spinal canal. Contrast MRI imaging shows spinal fluid as white.

Spacing: This refers to the normal space between cauda equina nerve roots as seen on axial MRI images. The space appears as white between gray or black nerve roots. Spacing disappears with nerve root enlargement or coalescence.

Spinal canal: Also known as the thecal sac. The spinal canal is a structure like a closed pipe that carries the spinal fluid. The fluid is primarily produced in the brain and flows down and up the canal to be diverted into head and neck lymph nodes and the general blood and lymphatic circulation. The word canal is preferentially used here to simplify understanding.

Symmetry and asymmetry: Cauda equina nerves normally free float in a symmetrical position with half on the right and half on left sides of the spinal canal. Asymmetry means that some nerve roots have been displaced or shifted from their normal position due to a disease process.

Thickening: Cauda equina nerve roots have a rather standard thickness. Thickening or enlargement means the roots have edema, inflammation, and/or scarring.

4. HOW LUMBAR SACRAL ADHESIVE ARACHNOIDITIS DEVELOPS

- Cauda equina nerve roots, which number about two dozen, hang downward and are suspended in spinal fluid. They are situated inside the spinal canal in a symmetrical right to left pattern with equal numbers on each side.

- AA occurs when a clump or group of cauda equina nerve roots become glued by adhesions to the inside of the spinal canal covering. Contrast MRIs can visualize this occurrence.[1,4,5,16,17]

- Normal frontal, lateral, and axial (toe-to-head) examples of cauda equina nerve roots are shown in this handbook. The tell-tale signs of chronic cauda equina nerve root inflammation include enlargement or thickening, loss of circular contour, and displacement from their normal, symmetrical position. When inflammation leads to adhesion formation, nerve roots begin to coalesce and clump. In the final stage nerve root clumps will glue to the inside of the spinal canal covering. The initial location or site of the inflammation can be in the arachnoid layer of the canal covering, or in the nerve roots.

- Once a clump of nerve roots develops due to inflammation and adhesions, fibrosus and calcification may occur and form a fibrotic tumor-like mass inside the spinal canal. This mass will interfere with and impair normal spinal fluid flow which may result in headaches, blurred vision, dizziness, poor balance, and tinnitus.[20]

5. FRONTAL ILLUSTRATION OF THE CAUDA EQUINA NERVE ROOTS

The cauda equina consists of about two dozen nerve roots that are suspended from the spinal cord which ends at about lumbar one-two (L1-L2). The roots are suspended in spinal fluid in a symmetrical position with half of them on the right and half on the left side of the spinal canal. The nerve roots exit the lumbar-sacral spinal canal beginning at the lower thoracic and upper lumbar regions, so there are fewer nerve roots in the lower lumbar and sacral regions than in the upper lumbar spinal canal.

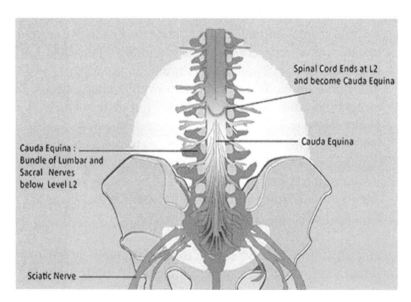

6. FRONTAL PHOTOGRAPH OF NORMAL CAUDA EQUINA NERVE ROOTS

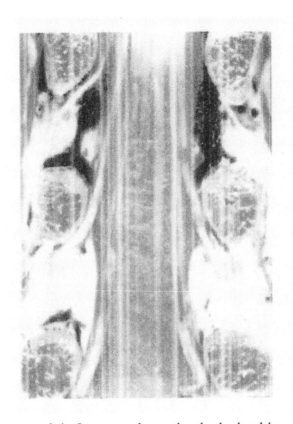

This photograph is from a cadaver that had a healthy spine. Note the end of the spinal cord at the top and the thin, "string like" character of the nerve roots.

7. LATERAL VIEW OF THE CAUDA EQUINA

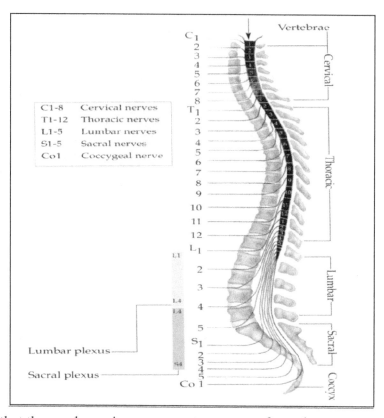

Note that the cauda equina nerve roots emanate from the lower thoracic and upper lumbar regions of the spinal cord. The nerve roots are freely suspended in spinal fluid. Some cauda equina nerve roots can become inflamed, develop adhesions, and adhere to the inside of the spinal canal covering. This is the essence of AA.

8. ANATOMICAL AXIAL APPEARANCE OF THE SPINAL CANAL

This view on an MRI is technically called the "axial" (toe-to-head) view.

NERVE ROOT POSITIONS ARE AT ABOUT L4-5

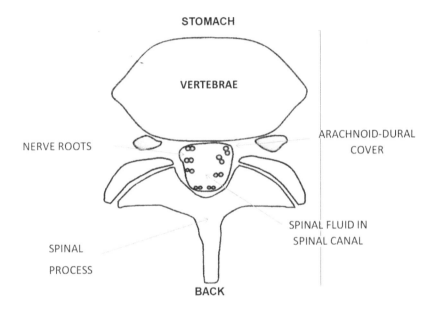

9. NORMAL POSITIONS OF THE CAUDA EQUINA NERVE ROOTS: AXIAL VIEWS

Shown here are maps of the nerve root positions at the various lumbar-sacral vertebral levels.[6,19] There are about two dozen nerve roots at L1-L2. The number of nerve roots decrease from L1-2 to L5-S1. Nerve roots are normally paired for ascending and descending neurons. There are equal numbers on each side of the canal. These position maps are generally evident on contrast MRIs and permit the differentiation of normal versus abnormal positioning of the cauda equina nerve roots. Note the relative circular contour and size of each nerve root. The nerve roots are spaced between each other and float freely in the spinal fluid.

Abnormalities visualized on contrast MRI of the cauda equina nerve roots include displacement, asymmetry, enlargement, loss of circular contour, and coalescence or clumping rather than the symmetrical, uniform, circular contour, and free-floating right and left positions of normal cauda equina nerve roots.

POSITION MAPS OF THE NERVE ROOTS

L_2-L_3

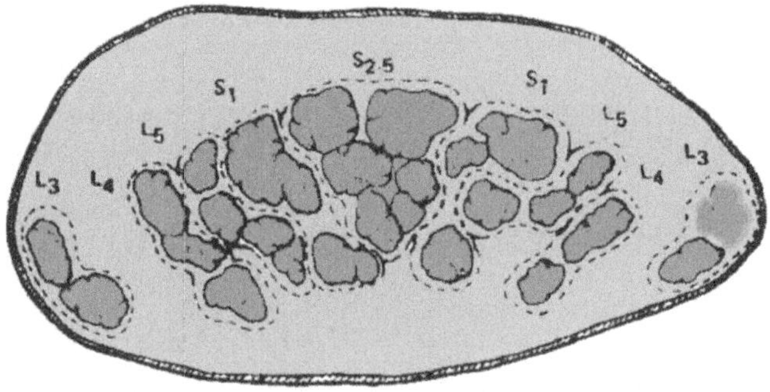

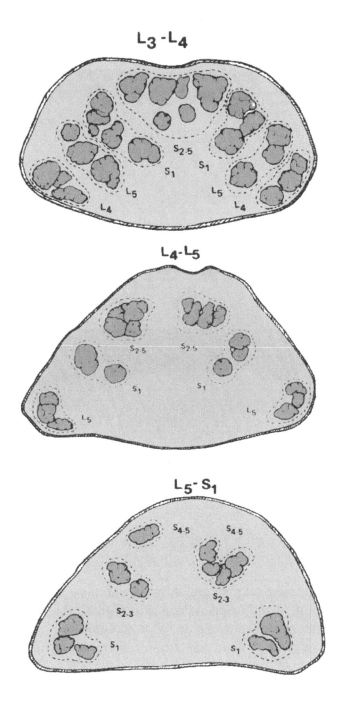

10. PHOTOGRAPHS OF NORMAL CAUDA EQUINA NERVE ROOTS: AXIAL VIEWS

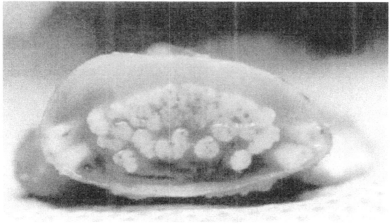

L1 - L3

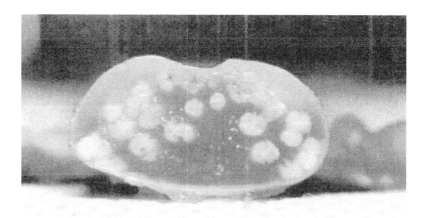

L3 – L4

The normal, symmetrical position of cauda equina nerve roots have been identified and mapped thanks to anatomical studies on cadavers that had a healthy spine.[6,19] Note in these examples the circular contour, relative size, and left and right symmetry of the nerve roots. There is clear space observed between nerve roots.

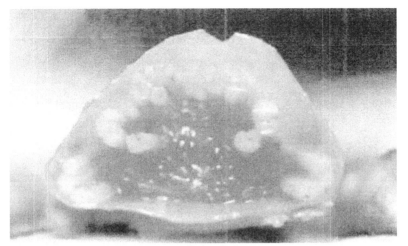

L4 – L5

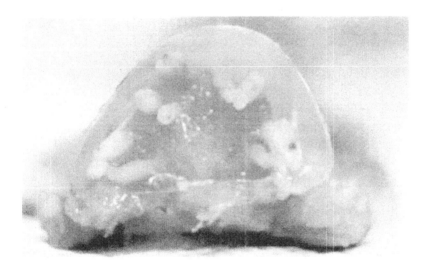

L5 – S1

11. NORMAL CONTRAST MRI IMAGE OF CAUDA EQUINA NERVE ROOTS: AXIAL VIEW

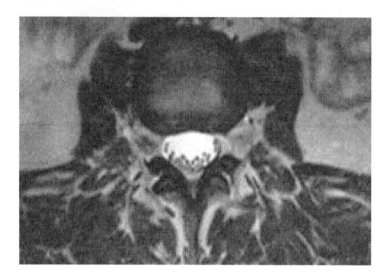

Note that the number of nerve roots are about equal on each side of the canal, and that they are in a symmetrical pattern. The nerve roots have a circular contour and are separated from each other. Clear space is observed between nerve roots. The level shown here is approximately L3-L4.

12. ABNORMALITIES FOUND ON AXIAL CONTRAST MRIs

The critical finding to diagnose AA is a clump of nerve roots that has become attached to the inside of the arachnoid-dural covering of the spinal canal.[1,2,4,7,14] Other findings suggestive of intraspinal canal inflammation and AA and include thickening and displacement of nerve roots. The circular contour of nerve roots may be erased or distorted. Normal canal shape may also be distorted and there may be thickening of the arachnoid-dural covering of the spinal canal suggestive of inflammation. There is a loss of space between nerve roots. A common and initiating finding in AA cases is the presence of intervertebral discs that protrude and press upon the spinal canal.[13]

Sometimes the determination that there is coalescence or clumping of nerve roots can be equivocal (or questionable) particularly in early or short-term cases. Late-stage AA clearly shows a loss of circular contour of nerve roots and clumping that may appear as a solid, dense fibrous mass. Calcification can occur in a mass of longstanding nature.[18]

Summary of Possible Abnormalities in Cauda Equina Nerve Roots

- ✓ Displacement and asymmetry
- ✓ Loss of visible space between nerve roots
- ✓ Enlargement/thickening
- ✓ Loss of circular contour
- ✓ Coalescence/clumping
- ✓ Mass/tumor formation
- ✓ Adherence of clumps to canal covering
- ✓ Calcification in clumps

13. ABNORMALITIES FOUND ON LATERAL CONTRAST MRIs

The lateral or sagittal view usually provides evidence of AA, as does the axial view. The major sign is called a "filling defect" next to the canal covering as the clumps or inflammatory adhesive masses don't allow spinal fluid to show next to the canal cover. Spinal fluid shows white on contrast MRI, and a normal spinal canal will show filling from the top to the bottom of the canal. The mass of AA may progress from one of inflammation and adhesions into a fibrous, dense scar which may even calcify.

In addition to filling defects the lateral view may show thickened bands of nerve roots, dilation of the canal, and the apparent absence of nerve roots in the lower lumbar-sacral spinal canal. This is known as the "empty sac" sign which is caused by adherence of cauda equina nerve roots to the inside of the spinal canal covering. This process is sometimes called peripheralization. The adherence of inflammatory clumps of nerve roots to the canal covering lowers the tensile strength of the arachnoid-dural covering so it appears as dilated on lateral MRI views.

The lateral view may also show perineural (Tarlov) cysts, and leakage or seepage of spinal fluid into tissues outside the spinal canal. We have observed what we believe to be a previously unreported sign, and that is tissue channels to the skin surface created by leaked or seeped spinal fluid that is attempting to escape. Skin contractures and indentions of the skin can sometimes be observed just over the area of the channels.

Summary of Possible Abnormalities
on Lateral View

- ✓ Mass or clump of nerve roots (non-filling defect)
- ✓ Band of thickened roots
- ✓ "Empty sac" – apparent absence of nerve roots
- ✓ Dilation of thecal sac (canal)
- ✓ Intervertebral discs pressing on canal
- ✓ Perineural (Tarlov) cysts
- ✓ Seepage of fluid outside spinal canal

14. BASIC APPEARANCE OF ADHESIVE ARACHNOIDITIS: SINGLE CLUMP

The basic appearance of AA is a clump of nerve roots that adheres by inflammatory adhesions to the inside of the spinal canal covering. Here is an example of a single clump in the spinal canal, that is adhered to the inside of the spinal canal covering.

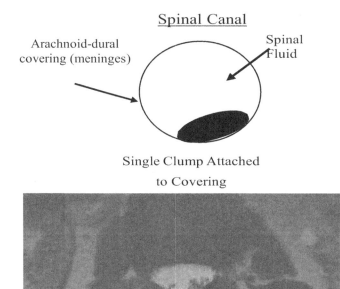

MRI image of single clump of nerve roots attached to the arachnoid-dural covering at about L4-L5. There may be thickening of the arachnoid-dural covering. Note that the nerve roots have lost their circular contour, are displaced to the right, and space between roots cannot be visualized.

15. BASIC APPEARANCE OF ADHESIVE ARACHNOIDITIS: MULTIPLE CLUMPS

Many clinical cases of AA show multiple clumps attached to the inside of the spinal canal covering on an axial contrast MRI.

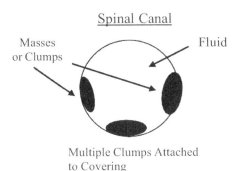

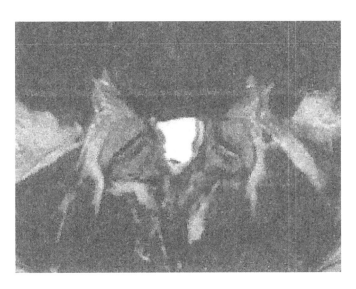

Note the distortion of the shape of the spinal canal and the multiple nerve root clumps that are adhered to the inside of the spinal canal cover. The clumps are dense as individual nerve roots cannot be identified. Tight adherence to the canal cover is sometimes called peripheralization. Note the lightened areas in the masses. This is likely calcification.

16. PROCESS AND TIME FRAME FOR DEVELOPMENT OF AA

AA is always caused by some initiating event or disease.[1,2,5,11] Consequently, it can usually be regarded as a secondary disorder or complication of another disease or disorder. The most common preceding disorder is inflamed intervertebral discs that protrude and press upon the spinal canal covering.[13] Trauma to the spinal canal covering by accident or medical procedure is also a common precipitating event. The time frame to develop AA following a protruding disc, infection, or autoimmune disease may range from months to years. We have, however been able to determine a general time frame from arachnoid-dural puncture to the visual presence of AA on contrast MRI. AA will not show on a contrast MRI for at least 4 to 8 weeks after an arachnoid-dural puncture. To develop AA there must first be inflammation in either the cauda equina or arachnoid-dural covering of the spinal canal. The original inflammation must fester, spread, and develop adhesions that glue the nerve roots to the canal cover. Prior to the development of AA a contrast MRI following a dural puncture may show enlargement, loss of circular contour, and asymmetry of nerve roots but no clumping of nerve roots. In our opinion, emergency treatment should be started if there are persisting clinical symptoms and some cauda equina abnormalities are present on MRI after a dural puncture. The hope is to prevent the development of AA.

AA Developmental Process
Following Arachnoid-Dural Puncture

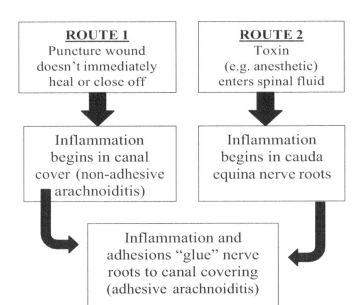

17. CLINICAL PROFILE OF ABNORMAL EXAMPLES

The examples of abnormal MRIs shown in this handbook are all from persons who had a majority of the following clinical manifestations and symptoms.

- ✓ Low back pain
- ✓ Pain periodically radiated into buttocks or legs
- ✓ Pain temporarily relieved upon standing or reclining
- ✓ Sensations of insects or dripping water on legs
- ✓ Burning sensation in feet or buttocks
- ✓ Pain on ascending stairs or straight leg raising
- ✓ Blurred vision, headaches, tinnitus, poor balance
- ✓ Dysfunction of bladder and/or bowel

It is not recommended that a search for AA by contrast MRI be done in a person without some typical symptoms of this disorder as we have no information on false negatives or positives.

It is not recommend simply to categorize clinical severity solely with MRI findings as they may not correlate.[11,15] Proper interpretation is to simply identify lower spinal canal nerve root abnormalities in a patient with typical symptoms of AA.

18. EXAMPLES OF NORMAL MRI AXIAL VIEWS

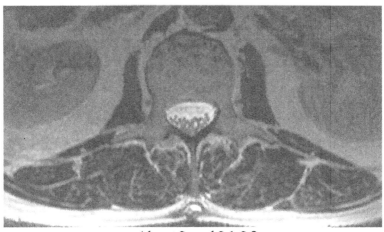

About Level L1-L2

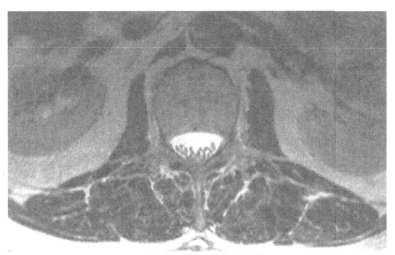

About Level L2-L3

Note the symmetry, size, circular contour, and spacing between nerve roots.

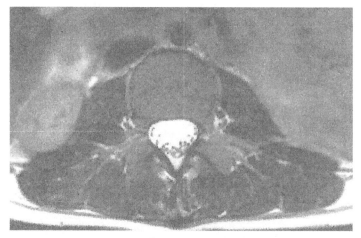

About Level L3-L4

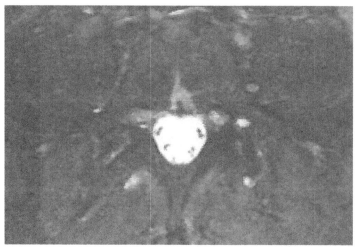

About Level L5-S1

19. EXAMPLES OF ABNORMAL AXIAL VIEW MRIs

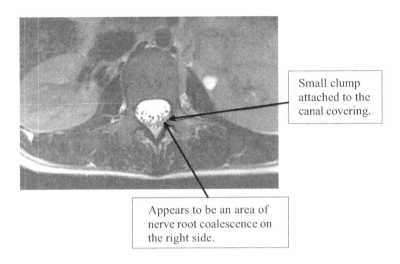

Small clump attached to the canal covering.

Appears to be an area of nerve root coalescence on the right side.

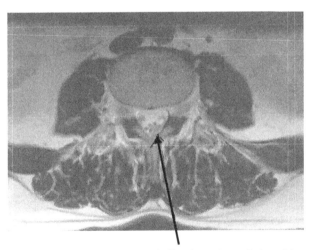

Nerve roots are enlarged and displaced to right. Clumping and attachment to the arachnoid-dural covering is evident.

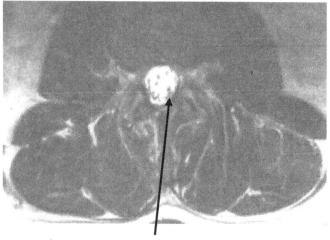

Nerve root clumps are adhered to the inside wall of the spinal canal.

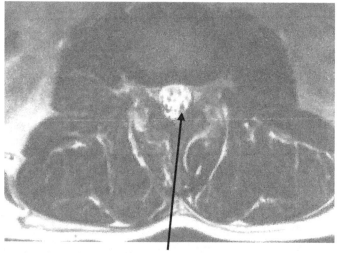

Gross disorganization, displacement, and asymmetry of nerve roots. Some have coalesced and lost their circular contour.

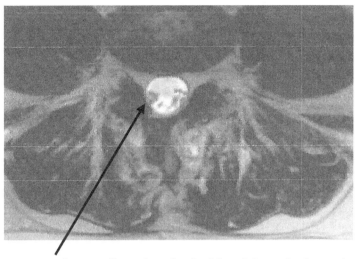

Nerve root clump adhered to the inside of the spinal canal.

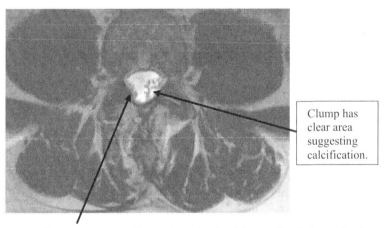

Clump has clear area suggesting calcification.

Mass of nerve roots adhered to the inside wall of the spinal canal.

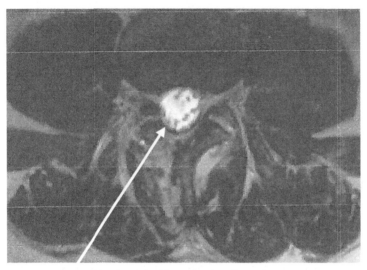

Nerve roots are displaced, disorganized, and have an asymmetrical pattern. Some are adhered to the inside wall of the spinal canal.

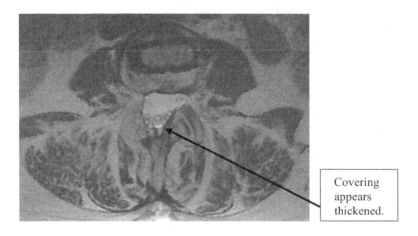

Covering appears thickened.

Shape of canal is distorted. Nerve roots have coalesced and lost their circular contour.

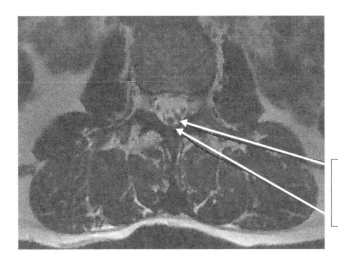

Multiple clumps of nerve roots.

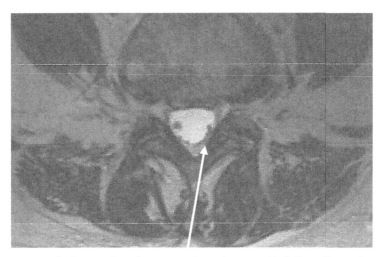

Nerve roots in lower lumbar-sacral region are tightly adhered to the spinal canal covering.

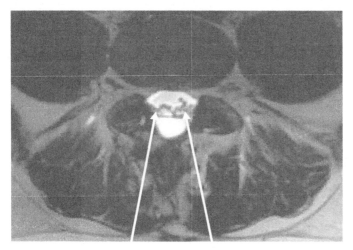

Shows severe AA – band of clumped roots – adhered on both ends to inside wall of the spinal canal. Calcification is apparent.

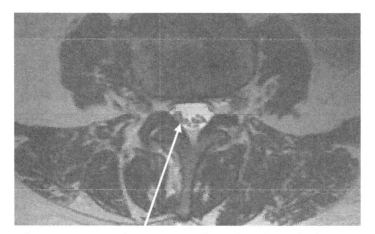

Clumps of nerve roots and some are adhered to the spinal canal covering by adhesions.

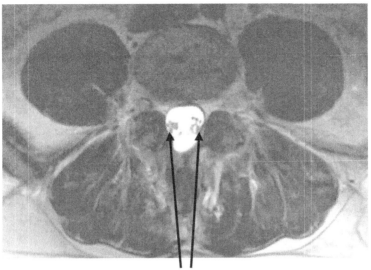

Nerve root clumping is on both sides of the spinal canal.

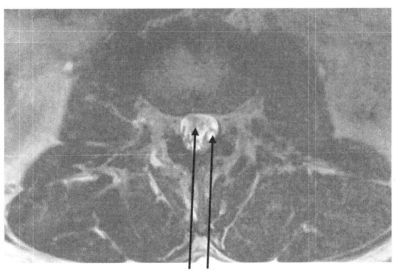

Essentially all nerve roots at about L2-L3 are involved in clump formation. Calcification is present.

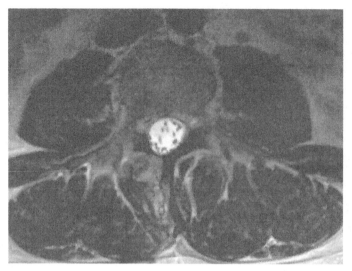

Nerve roots are displaced, asymmetrical in pattern, and some appear to be attached to the inside wall of the spinal canal.

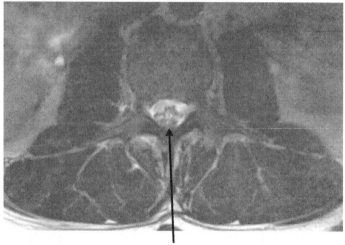

All nerve roots at about L2-3 are in a large, clumped mass. Calcification is present.

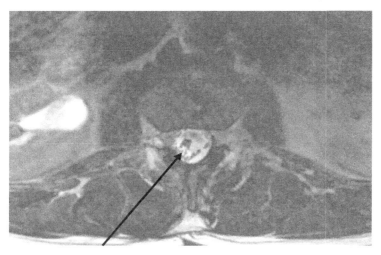

Multiple areas of clumping. Some are attached to the spinal canal covering.

Disc pressing against canal wall.

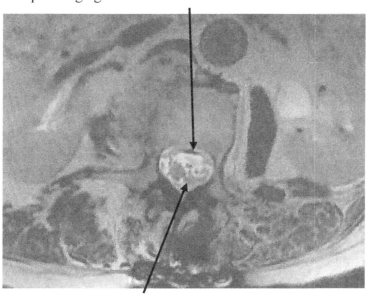

The inside of the spinal canal is filled with clumped, scarred nerve roots. Some calcification is present. Nerve roots have lost their circular contour.

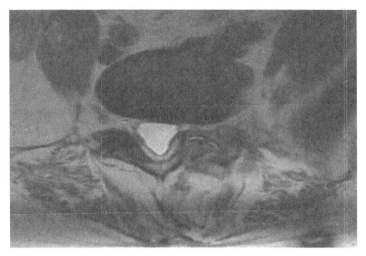

Empty sac appearance due to nerve roots being attached to the inside wall of the canal by adhesions.

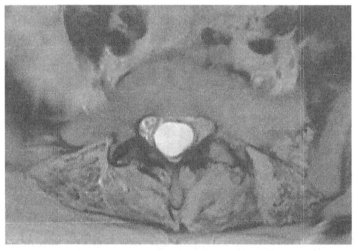

Empty sac appearance. The nerve roots in the sacral area are tightly adhered to the inside wall of the spinal canal.

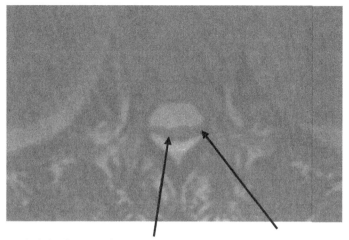

Scarred tight band of nerve roots is apparent. The band is attached to the canal covering at both ends.

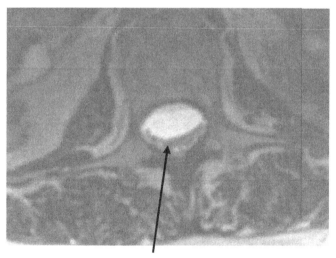

Thick band of essentially all nerve roots at about L4-L5. Scarring has resulted. No separate nerve roots can even be seen.

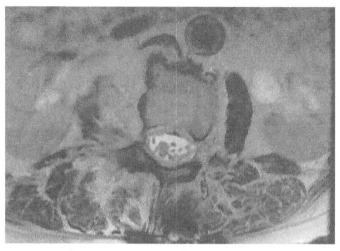

Multiple nerve root clumps at about L3-L4. Some are attached to the arachnoid-dural covering of the spinal canal.

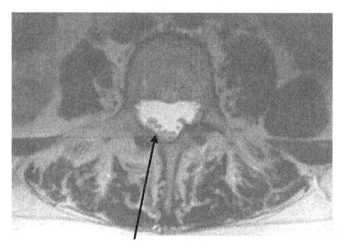

Cauda equina nerve roots have shifted to the left. Some nerve roots appear enlarged and have lost their circular contour. Attachment to the spinal canal wall is evident.

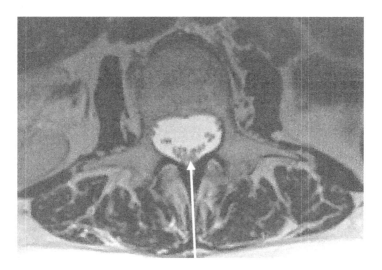

Nerve roots have clumped and are adhered to the inside of the spinal canal cover.

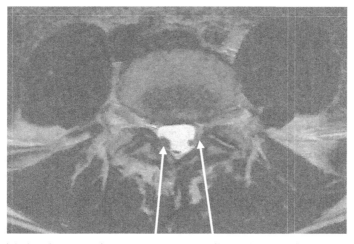

Multiple clumps of nerve roots are adhered to the inside of the arachnoid-dural covering of the spinal canal.

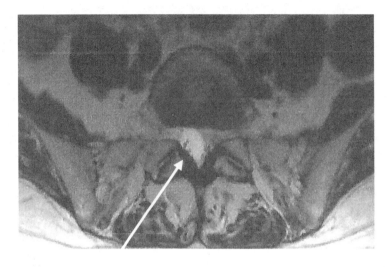

Distorted spinal canal. Thickened ligamentum flavum and spinal canal cover (meninges). Nerve roots are adhered to the canal cover.

20. NORMAL LATERAL VIEW MRI

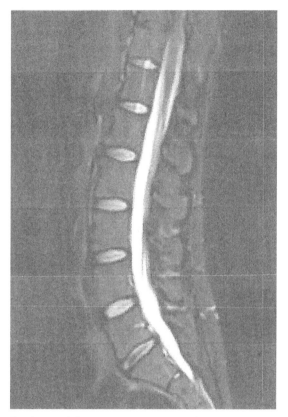

Normal spinal canal by contrast MRI. The white is spinal fluid. The gray or dark coloring inside the spinal canal are cauda equina nerve roots. Note that spinal fluid is present in a non-dilated canal, and it flows to the bottom of the sacral canal.

21. EXAMPLES OF ABNORMAL LATERAL VIEW MRIs

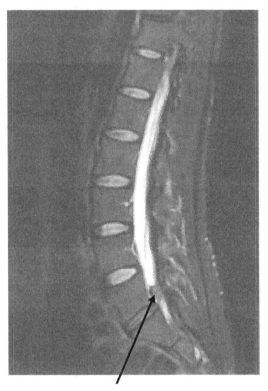

There is a mass of nerve roots that have resulted from inflammation and adhesions. There is adherence of the mass to the arachnoid-dural canal covering along with spinal fluid flow obstruction.

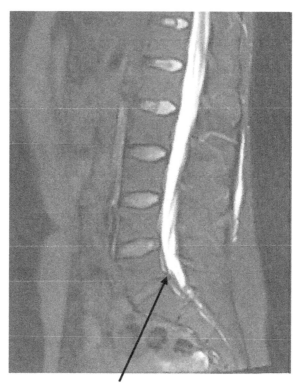

The disc at L4-S1 is pressing on the canal wall. There is a non-filling defect that is typical of an area of AA.

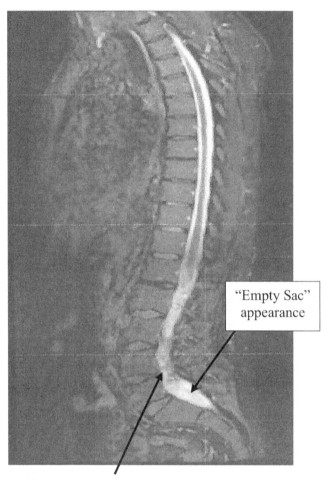

Poor filling due to fibrotic scarring.

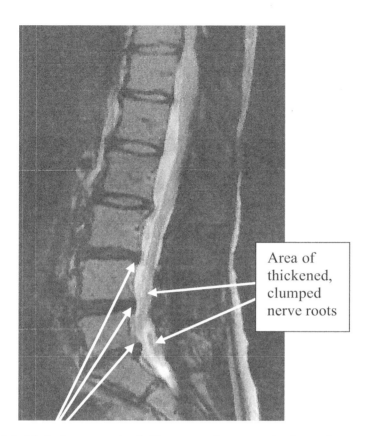

Multiple intervertebral discs pressing on spinal canal.

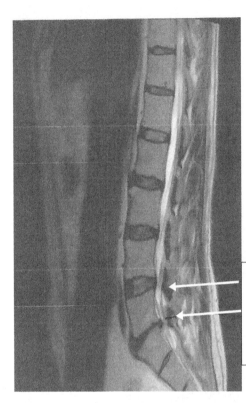

Filling defects which represent nerve roots that are inflamed and thickened.

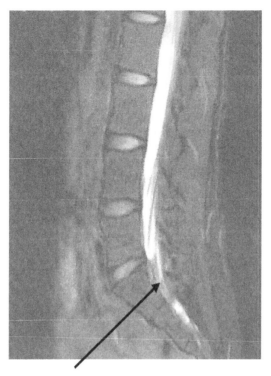

Filling defect just below L5-S1 disc that is pressing on the canal covering. Area is a mass of inflamed nerve roots adhered to the inside of the spinal canal by adhesions.

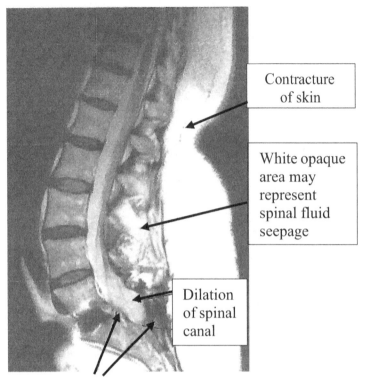

Areas of inflamed, clumped nerve roots that are likely scarred.

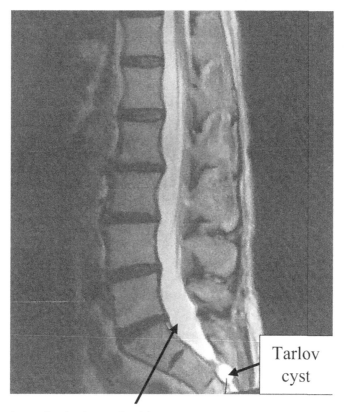

Dilation of spinal canal with "empty sac" appearance.

Handbook to Recognize Adhesive Arachnoiditis by (MRI)

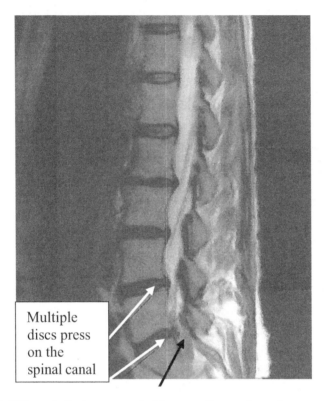

Fluid filling defects are probably scar tissue from long-standing inflammation and adhesion formation.

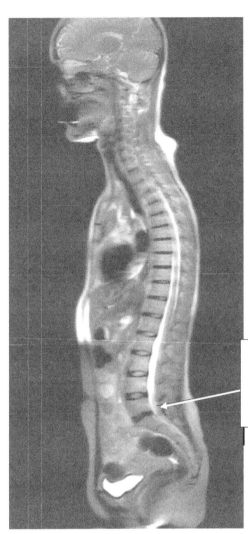

Filling defect that is area of thickened nerve roots. Spinal fluid flow channel is narrowed.

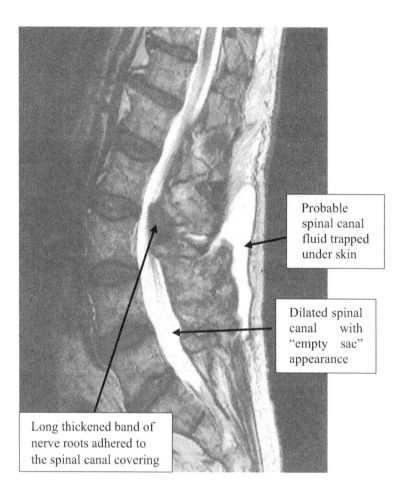

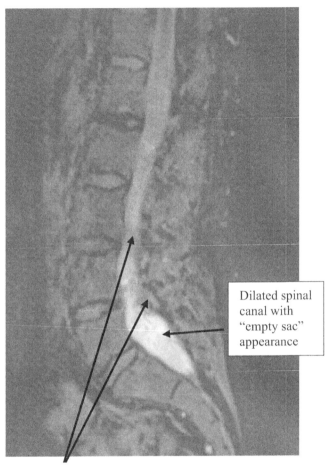

Filling defects due to fibrous masses of nerve roots attached to spinal canal cover.

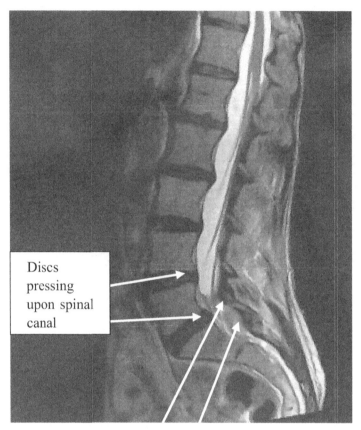

Non-filling defects that represent nerve root clumps, inflammation, and mass formation.

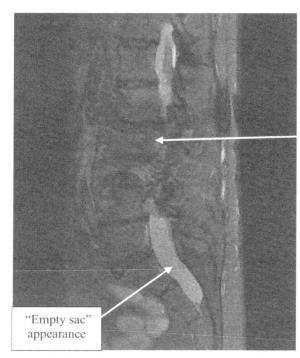

Spinal fluid flow is almost not visible due to the canal being filled with fibrotic, scarred nerve roots.

"Empty sac" appearance

22. SUMMARY

Adhesive arachnoiditis (AA) is an intraspinal, canal inflammatory disorder. It occurs when some cauda equina nerve roots become glued to the inside of the spinal canal covering due to inflammation and adhesions. The term arachnoid is applied because it is the layer of the spinal canal covering inside the outer, dural layer (meninges).

In 1909 the esteemed, British neurosurgeon, Sir Victor Horsley, operated on and described 21 cases of what today would be called "Adhesive Arachnoiditis." [12] He originally believed all his cases had a spinal canal tumor as they had pain and varying degrees of paraplegia. During his surgeries he found the spinal canal to be distended and to contain a considerable amount of excess fluid. Nerve roots were edematous and "matted." The arachnoid-dural canal covering was inflamed often for several inches in length. He found it necessary to perform a laminectomy in every case.

Today all of Dr. Horsley's findings can now be observed on the new, contrast MRIs. Furthermore, these MRI findings can be easily observed by a medical practitioner who spends a little time to study how to interpret MRIs in a person with typical symptoms of AA. This handbook is an end-result of reviewing over, 600 MRIs of persons with AA. The purpose of the handbook is to encourage medical practitioners to recognize AA as early as possible so humanitarian treatment can be initiated.

REFERENCES

1. Aldrete JA. History and evaluation of arachnoiditis: The evidence revealed. *Insurgentes Centro 51-A. Col San Rafael, Mexico* 2010; p3-14.
2. Anderson TL, Morris JM, Wald JT, et al. Imaging appearance of advanced chronic adhesive arachnoiditis: A retrospective review. *Asr Am J Roentgenol* 2017;209:648-655.
3. Bilello J, Tennant F. Patterns of chronic inflammation in extensively treated patients with arachnoiditis and chronic intractable pain. *Postgrad Med* 2016;92(17):1-5.
4. Bourne IH. Lumbo-sacral adhesive arachnoiditis: A review. *J R Soc Med* 1990;83:262-265.
5. Burton C. Lumbosacral arachnoiditis. *Spine* 1978;3:24-30.
6. Cohen MS, Wall EJ, Kerber CW, et al. The anatomy of the cauda equina on CT scans and MRI. *J Bone Joint* Surg 1991;73-B:381-384.
7. Delamarter RB Ross JS, Masaryk TS, etal. Diagnosis of lumbar arachnoiditis by magnetic resonance imaging. *Spine* 1990;15:304-310.
8. Eisenberg E, Goldman R, Schlag-Eisenberg D, Grinfeld A. Adhesive arachnoiditis following lumbar epidural steroid injections: A report of two cases and review of literature. *J Pain Research* 2019;12:513- 518.
9. Harvey SC. Meningeal adhesions and their significance. *Interstate Post Grad Med, North America Prac* 1926;2:27-31.
10. Henderson FC, Austin C, Benzel E, et al. Neurological and spinal manifestations of the Ehlers-Danlos Syndromes. *Amer J Men Gen* 2017;175C:195-211.
11. Homsi ME, Gharzeddine K, Cuevas J, et al. MRI findings of arachnoiditis revisited: Is classification possible? *J Morgan Rason Imaging* 2021;DOI:10.1002/jmri.27583.
12. Horsley V. Chronic spinal meningitis: its differential diagnosis and surgical treatment. *Br J Med* 1909;1:513-517.
13. Jackson A, Isherwood I. Does degenerative disease of the lumbar spine cause arachnoiditis? A magnetic resonance study and review ofthe literature. *Brit J Radiology* 1994;67:840-847.
14. Jorgenson J, Hansen PH, Steenskoo V, et al. A clinical and radiological study of chronic lower spinal arachnoiditis. *Neuroradiology* 1975;9:139-144.
15. Parenti V, Huda F, Richardson PK, et al. Lumbar arachnoiditis: Does imaging associate with clinical features? *Clin Neurol Neurosurg* 2020;192:105717.
16. Quiles M, Marchiselo PJ, Tsairis P. Lumbar adhesive arachnoiditis:Etiologic and pathologic aspects. *Spine* 1978;3:45-50

17. Ross JS, Masaryk TS, Modic MT, et al. MRI imaging of lumbar arachnoiditis. *A J R Am J* Roentgenol 1987;149:1025-1032.
18. Shiraish T, Crook HV, Reynolds A. Spinal arachnoiditis ossificans: Observations on its investigation and treatment. *European Spine* J 1995;4:60-63.
19. Wall, Chohen MS, Abithal JJ, et al. Organization of intrathecal nerve roots at the level of conus medularis. J Bone Joint Surg *1990;72:1495-1499.*
20. Whendon JM, Glassey D. Cerebrospinal fluid stasis and its clinical significance. *Altern Ther Health Med* 2009;15(3):54-60.

INDEX

adherence, 20, 23, 44
adhesive arachnoiditis, 1, 59
axial views, 14, 16, 27
burning, 5, 26
cadaver, 11
calcification, 6, 9, 23, 37
cauda equina, 1, 3, 5, 6, 8, 9, 10, 12, 14, 16, 20, 24, 43, 59
circular contour, 6, 9, 14, 16, 18, 19, 22, 24, 27, 30, 32, 37, 40
coalescence, 6, 8, 14, 19
contrast, 3, 5, 6, 8, 9
disease, 2, 5, 8, 24
disorganization, 30
displacement, 7, 9, 14, 19, 30
Ehlers Danlos Syndrome, 3
empty sac, 7, 20, 51
fibrosus, 9
Harvey, Samuel, 2
Horsley, Victor, 2, 59
inflammation, 1, 2, 3, 5, 6, 8, 9, 19, 20, 24, 44, 52, 56, 59
intervertebral discs, 3, 5, 19, 24, 47
lumbar spine, 61
Lyme, 3
magnetic resonance imaging, 1
maps, 14

mass, 5, 6, 9, 19, 20, 36, 44, 49, 56
meninges, 2, 3, 6, 7, 22, 42, 59
nerve root, 5, 7, 8, 9, 14, 23, 26, 40, 56
pain, 1, 2, 3, 5, 14, 26, 59
perineural, 20
peripheralization, 23
puncture, 24
sacral, 3, 4, 5, 7, 10, 14, 20, 33, 38, 43
seepage, 20
spacing, 27
spinal canal, 1, 2, 3, 4, 5, 6, 7, 8, 9, 10, 12, 19, 20, 21, 22, 23, 24, 26, 30, 31, 32, 33, 34, 35, 36, 37, 38, 40, 41, 42, 43, 47, 49, 51, 55, 59
spinal cord, 2, 6, 10, 11, 12, 19
spinal fluid, 2, 3, 6, 7, 8, 9, 10, 12, 14, 20, 43, 44
spine, 3, 4, 7, 11, 16
symmetry, 16, 27
symptoms, 1, 5, 6, 26
thecal sac, 8, 21
thoracic spine, 4, 6, 10, 12
tumor, 9, 19, 59
urination, 5

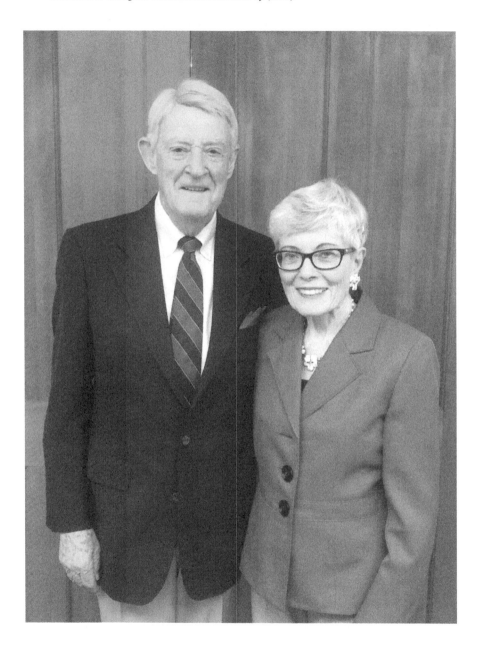

About The Author

Forest Tennant has spent most of his medical career as a practicing physician and researcher in the fields of addiction and pain medicine. He has published over 300 scientific articles and books in these fields. For his efforts he was recently given a "50 Year Achievement" award by "Pain Week." In this 50-year span he has been a US Army Medical Officer, UCLA Professor, Public Health Physician, Drug Advisor for the Los Angeles Dodgers, NASCAR, and the National Football League. He was editor of Practical Pain Management for 12 years. He recently retired from clinical practice to do research on intractable pain and the spinal cord disorder known as arachnoiditis. He and his wife, Miriam, have been married 55 years and they split their residence between West Covina, California and Wichita, Kansas, where they headquarter their real-estate company, Tennant Homes. Their charitable giving and medical research are sponsored by the Tennant Foundation.

Other Books by Forest Tennant

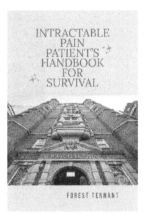

"Intractable Pain Patients Handbook for Survival"
ISBN:9781955934121
LOC:2021916464

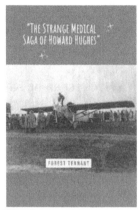

"THE STRANGE MEDICAL SAGA
OF HOWARD HUGHES"
ISBN: 9781955934091
LOC: 2021912855

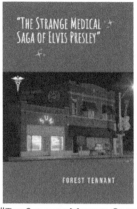

"THE STRANGE MEDICAL SAGA
OF ELVIS PRESLEY"
ISBN: 9781955934008
LOC: 2021911718

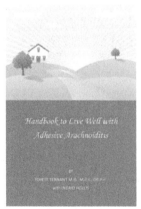

"HANDBOOK TO LIVE WELL WITH ADHESIVE
ARACHNOIDITIS"
ISBN: 978195934060
LOC: 2021912718

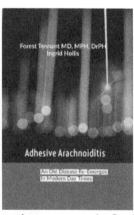

"ADHESIVE ARACHNOIDITIS: AN OLD DISEASE
RE-EMERGES IN MODERN TIMES"
ISBN: 9781955934039
LOC: 2021912467

Made in the USA
Las Vegas, NV
11 February 2025